I0413402

Apple Cider Vinegar:

Health Benefits and Precautions

By

Debra Helton

ISBN-13: 978-1495920899

Table of Contents

Apple Cider Vinegar: Health Benefits and Precautions

By Debra Helton

© Copyright 2013 Debra Helton

Reproduction or translation of any part of this work beyond that permitted by section 107 or 108 of the 1976 United States Copyright Act without permission of the copyright owner is unlawful. Requests for permission or further information should be addressed to the author.

This publication is designed to provide accurate and authoritative information in regard to the subject matter covered. This work is sold with the understanding that the publisher is not engaged in rendering legal, accounting, or other professional services. If legal advice or other expert assistance is required, the services of a competent professional person should be sought.

First Published, 2013

Printed in the United States of America

1. Introduction

At this point, you must've heard about apple cider vinegar. Everybody's crossed paths with this amazing creation at one point or another.

But what does it do? How does it help you?

Are there any health benefits and precautions that I need to be aware of?

If you have been asking yourself any of the questions above, then you are wise beyond your years. It's good to know the health benefits and information about all kinds of products and health-related items.

That's why I'd like to share much of today's leading information in regards to apple cider vinegar and all that it can do for you.

You see, the health benefits and precautions for this type of vinegar are numerous. Thankfully, the health benefits are numerous and the precautions are few. But you need to know both sides of the story in order to enjoy the amazing healthy benefits that this type of vinegar can provide.

So, in an effort to further enlighten you, I think it would be helpful to share the health benefits, precautions, side effects and pertinent information about this excellent health source.

Let's get into the major details without any further delay...

2. Are You Using Apple Cider Vinegar As a Cure for Acne?

To start things off, I wanted to mention that using apple cider vinegar is an excellent way to treat acne. If you've never tried it before, then you are about to learn an exceptional way to eliminate unwanted acne once and for all.

This is an outstanding product for the skin. It is great at the detoxifying and cleansing your body and the health benefits are widespread. Apple cider vinegar has consistently provided great results for acne treatment, and there haven't been any negative side effects in this regard.

Why is apple cider vinegar so great at eliminating acne?

It contains natural properties that instantly fight against this condition. It has detoxifying properties, purification properties and cleansing properties.

Certain forms of acne are caused by the presence of free radicals. Other forms of acne are caused due to harmful toxins permeating your skin. These harmful toxins usually occur due to improper diet.

When you use apple cider vinegar to treat unwanted acne, it will balance your body and eliminate the harmful toxins and free radicals that are negatively affecting your skin. You should certainly give it a try if you have unwanted acne ruining your complexion.

Let's see what else Apple cider vinegar can do...

3. Apple Cider Vinegar Can Remove Unwanted Warts

Yes, you read that correctly. Do you have any unwanted warts blemishing your otherwise beautiful skin? Have you tried other remedies to eliminate these warts, but nothing seems to work.

Well, it's time to give apple cider vinegar a try.

There is a simple method that you can use to kill any unwanted wart. Let's take a look at the method right now, so you can use it and cleanse your body of this unwanted condition.

For starters, you have to pick up apple cider vinegar from the local grocery store. If you can't find it there for some reason, then go to a health food store in your neighborhood. They will definitely carry it.

Next, you need to pour a half of cup of vinegar and mix it with a cup of warm water. The ratio is two parts water to one part apple cider vinegar. You need to dilute this solution so that it does not damage the healthy areas of your skin.

Third, it's time to soak your warts. So please make sure that you immerse your wart into the mixture and leave it there for a total of 20 minutes each day. After about a week's time, the wart should have been completely removed. It will slowly diminish in size after each soaking.

Here's a bonus method that I'd like to share...

Fully soak a cotton ball in apple cider vinegar. Next, take that cotton ball and tape it or fasten it over the wart so that it stays in place. You want to cover the wart with the soaked cotton ball overnight, and leave it there while you are sleeping.

This will also take about a week to work, but it's easier than spending 20 minutes a day soaking your wart in the vinegar solution provided above.

Next up on our list...

4. Apple Cider Vinegar Is Excellent for Weight Loss and Improved Digestion

In this day and age, with the average American diet haunting so many people, weight loss and digestion issues are running rampant throughout the world.

Even though I mention the average American diet, the American fast food lifestyle is spreading all throughout the world. So what was once known as the American diet is slowly becoming the fast food diet known and utilized all around the world.

It may make our lives easier to eat fast food all the time, but at what cost? We're damaging your health and shortening our lives all at the same time.

But here's the great thing...

Apple cider vinegar can help your body lose those unwanted pounds and get your digestion back on track once again.

One of the reasons why people are overweight is poor digestion. When a person suffers from digestive issues, their body no longer breaks down proteins and fats properly. This in turn causes the person with digestive issues to gain lots of weight and have a difficult time shedding the pounds.

When you take apple cider vinegar, it can help restore your body's acid levels to their normal state of being. So, your body will be able to digest food a lot easier, and it will do so more thoroughly.

This in turn will allow your body to absorb nutrients properly, and nutrient absorption is essential to overall health and well-being.

Another great thing about apple cider vinegar is that it helps you feel fuller when you take it.

So, you will eat a lot less and you'll have a lot less food to digest and break down.

So you'll naturally put yourself on a healthier diet by eating less, and your body will break down the food better and absorb the nutrients properly. That sounds like a win-win situation to me, and an excellent reason to start taking apple cider vinegar every day.

You will be able to get a slimmer, trimmer and healthier body when you use apple cider vinegar for weight loss. ACV is known to speed up the body's metabolism; it is known that when the body's metabolism is increased, he is more likely to lose more weight. It is recommended that anyone that would like to improve his metabolism drink ACV. Mix 2 teaspoons of vinegar in about an 8 ounce glass of water and then drink this mixture before he takes his meals. This will speed up his metabolism allowing the body to easily digest the food that he will eat and thus prevent accumulating extra weight and unsightly fat in the long run.

5. Apple Cider Vinegar Can Help Prevent Cancer

I know this may seem hard to believe for some of you, but it is widely known that this type of vinegar is able to slow the growth of cancer cells.

There have been studies that show that apple cider vinegar could possibly even kill cancer cells altogether. But I'd like to make one thing very clear...

Some of the results of these studies have been contradictory. So this is a subject under much discussion. If you are suffering from cancer, it certainly couldn't hurt to try apple cider vinegar to see if it has any positive effects.

There's nothing wrong with attempting to test this alternative treatment along with the other treatments mentioned and recommended by your doctor.

For all you know, apple cider vinegar may end up being the answer to your prayers. That's certainly an excellent reason to give it a try in my book. I surely hope you agree.

Here are a few reasons why people believe apple cider vinegar is capable of fighting cancer...

Some say that the acetic acid found in the vinegar is the actual cancer fighting ingredient. Other people believe that the pectin found in apples, along with the polyphenols, is the potential cancer fighting agents.

As of the time of this writing, it is still a mystery as to what causes apple cider vinegar to arrest the development of cancer. Just know that it has been effective for some, so it certainly may be affective for you.

You'll never know unless you give it a try. So that's exactly what I suggest you do.

Moving on to the next topic of our discussion...

6. Can Apple Cider Vinegar Help Improve Blood Pressure and Cholesterol Levels?

The next excellent discovery that I'd like to bring to your attention is apple cider vinegar's ability to significantly reduce cholesterol levels. But there's one caveat that you must be aware of...

When this study was originally done, it was performed on rats. So, there are people that speculate that it may not be able to perform the same way in humans.

More studies need to be completed in order to confirm the benefits of apple cider vinegar and lowering cholesterol in human beings.

A similar study was done on human beings in regards to blood pressure levels. The results were very positive when it came to lowering blood pressure, and apple cider vinegar was also linked to reducing the risks of heart disease.

Since apple cider vinegar has such few side effects, taking a regular dose of it every day is excellent if you're looking to reduce heart disease. So that's certainly something to think about in regards to your health.

7. Can Apple Cider Vinegar Help Detoxify the Liver and Other Bodily Organs?

This form of vinegar contains antibacterial properties. These properties are excellent for cleansing the body of toxic buildup and harmful bacteria.

Human beings function at their best when their body's pH balance is at optimal levels. You need to stabilize these levels in order to feel healthy and strong.

Taking a regular dose of apple cider vinegar will promote the natural cleansing effect inside of your body. It's also a great way to treat any allergies that you may have, and you can use it to clean mucus out of your sinuses. It's also great at cleansing your lymph nodes.

The best way to take apple cider vinegar for detoxification purposes is to buy organic, unpasteurized and unfiltered forms of this product. It's even recommended that you purchase untreated vinegar in order to maximize the health benefits available to you.

Just remember to take his wonderful product every day, and it will certainly help cleanse your body, detox your liver and release unwanted toxins and harmful bacteria from your organs.

Let's now move on to the side effects and safety precautions that you must learn about apple cider vinegar...

8. Other Health Benefits

8.1 Gastrointestinal Problems

Apple cider vinegar contains the substance called pectin and this helps ease a variety of gastrointestinal problems like diarrhea, spasms and colic. ACV is a natural treatment for these conditions; one or two tablespoons of vinegar in an 8 ounce glass of water would calm down an aching tummy. You may also try taking apple cider vinegar with fruit juice or apple juice if you find it intolerable to drink ACV with plain water.

8.2 Hiccup Control

Hiccups are known to be caused by eating a large meal in such a short period of time, slow digestion time of proteins or it may be due to low amounts of stomach acid. Apple cider vinegar is acid and can return the normal pH of the gastrointestinal system which may be able to reduce hiccups. By drinking 2 tablespoons of ACV in a glass of water for two times a day, you will be able to reduce gastric irritation and return the pH of the stomach. This will help reduce chronic hiccups and spasms of the gastrointestinal system.

8.3 Remove Nasal Stuffiness

When you have a cold you simply cannot breathe through the nose and this could cause major discomfort especially before you sleep. Drinking 2 teaspoons of apple cider vinegar in an 8 ounce glass of water will quickly help you breathe through your nose. You may sip this little by little until you have regained breathing through your nose.

8.4 Sore Throat

Sore throat or pain and irritation felt over the throat or neck area may be due to bacteria. Aside from pain over the area, there are also symptoms like fever, cough, nasal stuffiness and severe discomfort felt all over the body. Apple cider vinegar will help kill germs that cause sore throat since there are bacteria that will never survive an acidic environment. Take about ¼ cup of apple cider vinegar in ¼ cup of warm water and then gargle. You will feel a lot better after you use ACV as a gargle but you need to repeat this at every hour to kill bacteria effectively.

8.5 Swelling Reduce

Edema is the term to describe the swelling of any limb and in pregnancy; the most common areas that are prone to swelling are the feet, legs and the hands. Warm your hands by rubbing them together or by clapping them together and use about one to two tablespoons of ACV. Place vinegar on your palms and apply on the swelling. Apply long massage strokes on the area starting from the top most part of the leg to the lowest part. If the swelling is on the feet, you may soak your feet in a small basin of warm water with apple cider vinegar. Soak them for about 15 to 20 minutes and then wipe dry. Lie down with your legs or feet higher than the body to reduce swelling.

For swelling due to inflammation you may also apply apple cider vinegar on the affected area by using the same method. For swelling of the gums or mucous membranes, gargle apple cider vinegar in a glass of warm water.

Concentrate the mixture on the swelling and then rinse. Follow up with a gargle of warm water.

8.6 Remove Bad Breath

Bad breath may be due to so many reasons. It may be because of poor oral hygiene, dental caries, gastrointestinal problems and it may also be due to the food that you just ate. But regardless of the reason for bad breath apple cider vinegar may help. Gargle apple cider vinegar about 2 tablespoons in a tall glass of water after you wake up or after eating a meal with very strong flavors. Gargle this solution after every meal to ensure that the mouth is clean and free from bits of foods that can cause tooth decay. Apple cider vinegar is highly acidic and therefore will destroy bacteria that causes bad breath. Be sure to swish it in the mouth and to gargle with clean water afterwards.

8.7 Yeast Killer

The human body naturally has small amounts of fungus in different parts of the body like the skin, mucous membranes and the gastrointestinal system. Yeast often increases in number when the natural organisms like bacteria in the area reduce in number. A full-blown yeast infection happens when yeast multiply at an alarming rate. Apple cider vinegar is an acid and acid kills yeast. Therefore ACV will work well reducing yeast infection.

For oral yeast infection, use a few drops of pure ACV. Dip a cotton tip applicator in vinegar and apply it directly on the sore. Repeat this for about three times a day. You may also gargle 2 teaspoons of vinegar in an 8 ounce glass.

For yeast infections of the gastrointestinal system, drink apple cider vinegar in warm water. Mix 2 tablespoons of ACV in an 8 ounce glass. If you cannot tolerate this, take ACV with fruit juice or apple juice. Drink this once in the morning.

For yeast infections of the vagina or penile area, prepare a douche using a few tablespoons of apple cider vinegar in a small basin of warm water. Use this mixture as a douche. Use it at least twice or thrice a day.

In all cases of yeast infection symptoms must be followed closely. Treatment of yeast infection using ACV needs to be combined with aggressive measures like antifungal treatments to be able to completely resolve yeast infections.

8.8 Hair Care

When you shampoo and use styling products every day you tend to accumulate product residues on your scalp which makes hair dull and could cause irritation of the scalp. The acetic acid in apple cider vinegar will help remove this build up and make hair shinier and full of health. The best way to use ACV is to dilute about 1/3 cup into 4 cups of warm water. After shampooing using a regular brand of shampoo, rinse and then pour the vinegar and water solution on your hair; allow this to stand for about 15 minutes and then rinse. Use this treatment at least once a week to ensure that your scalp and hair strands are clean.

8.9 Skin Care

Just like the scalp, skin on the body and on the face tend to accumulate all kinds of residue, dirt and oils after exposure to pollution and the use of various skin care products. A special face mask may be used to remove dirt and oil on the face: use a part apple cider vinegar, bentonite clay and about a tablespoon of honey. Mix these ingredients really well in a small bowl and then apply to a clean face. Allow to remain on skin for about 15 minutes and then rinse using warm water. Repeat this treatment once a week.

For toning the skin, use plain apple cider vinegar on a cotton ball. Apply on dry skin or flaking skin; rub on the affected area using small circular strokes. Use a cotton ball with apple cider vinegar and apply on the dry areas of your face like the T-zone over the nose and forehead. Use this treatment at least once a day before going to sleep; this will minimize breakouts and blemishes on the area.

For treating the dry and dull skin in various areas of the body, you may place half a cup of apple cider vinegar into a tub-full of warm water. Soak for at least 20 minutes. Not only will you have healthy and radiant skin but will also draw out toxins from the body. Indulge in this moisturizing treatment every night just before you retire.

8.10 Teeth Care

A teaspoon of apple cider vinegar in warm water will make an effective gargle. This will remove not just bits of food that can cause tooth decay but will also make breath smell better and fresher longer. AVC will also make a great teeth whitener. Gargle ACV and water every day after brushing your teeth.

8.11 Foot Care

Your feet deserve a lot of attention after you get home from work or after a tiring day. Aside from just using soapy warm water to soak them use a mixture of warm water and half a cup of apple cider vinegar. Soak your feet for about 15 to 20 minutes and then pat dry with a soft towel. ACV will soothe swelling and will deodorize your feet. You may use this relaxing foot soak every time you come home or with a pumice stone, rub the rough skin on the soles of your feet like a foot spa every weekend.

8.12 Defy Aging

Apple cider vinegar is known to have anti-aging properties. It can minimize pores, remove blemishes and tone skin after regular use. After washing your skin, apply AVC using a cotton ball on the dry and blemished areas of your face. Let the vinegar stay on skin; repeat this every day. For tough and dry areas of the skin like the elbows, knees and ankles, rub pure ACV to reduce dryness and make your skin look younger and softer.

8.13 Sun Protection

The harsh UVB rays of the sun will make your skin dull, blemished and old. You may use apple cider vinegar on skin to treat sun burns and dull spots due to frequent exposure to the sun's rays. Use ACV in a cotton ball and simply dab it on the areas that you want to treat. Use this treatment every day. The best way to reduce exposure to the sun is the use of sunblock with SPF 50+. Do not attempt to go out under the sun without any protection.

8.14 Deodorant

Apple cider vinegar is a natural deodorizer and will remove smells and stains on clothes as well as on skin. Use a cotton ball with ACV and apply over the armpit and let dry. ACV will remove irritating body odor but will stain clothes so you must dry the armpit completely before wearing colored shirts.

Aside from removing embarrassing underarm odor, it will also reduce dark spots of the underarms and other folds of the skin. Regular use will never dry out skin or irritate skin but will improve the color of the underarms a few shades whiter.

8.15 Reduce Arthritis Symptoms

Arthritis could be very painful and may lead to decreased use of the extremity affected with arthritis. Apple cider vinegar may help; it is rich in minerals that can reduce joint pains. Magnesium, calcium, potassium and phosphorous are minerals that are either absent or reduced in the diet of a person suffering from arthritis. Potassium for one prevents the accumulation of calcium deposits in the joints that causes pain, weakening and swelling.

The ideal way to take apple cider vinegar is about a tablespoon just before eating. You may also mix 2 to 3 teaspoons of AVC in a glass of water and then drink before every meal (breakfast, lunch and dinner). If you cannot tolerate this mixture, place ACV in apple juice or add Stevia to sweeten the mixture instead. You may also rub pure apple cider vinegar over the affected joint just like rubbing mineral oil.

You may also soak the affected foot or hand in apple cider vinegar and warm water bath. Place half a cup of AVC in a small basin of warm water and soak for at least 20 minutes.

9. Side Effects and Safety Concerns of Apple Cider Vinegar

To start this section off, I'd like to point out that taking apple cider vinegar in food proportions is likely a safe thing to do. If you use this for medical purposes in the short term, it shouldn't cause any harm whatsoever.

As a matter of fact, it should help improve your health for the purposes in which you plan to use it.

But, there are instances when consuming large amounts of apple cider vinegar will not be safe. If you were to consume 8 ounces of the substance each day, and do it on a long-term basis, it could potentially lead to low potassium levels throughout your body.

There is one report which shows us that a person taking apple cider vinegar on a long-term basis developed osteoporosis and low potassium levels. The person was taking 250 mL of this substance daily, and they did it for 6 years.

Now let's take a look at the warnings and special precautions that you must be aware of...

9.1 Diabetes

The good thing about apple cider vinegar is that it's capable of lowering your blood sugar levels. This is a very good thing if you have diabetes. The warning is here because you need to monitor your levels very closely, because you may need to adjust your medication. Other than that, there's nothing to worry about as a diabetic.

9.2 Breast-feeding and pregnancy

We do not have enough information about apple cider vinegar at this point. If you are pregnant and plan to breast-feed, it's best to avoid this food source during this time.

Summary

I hope you found this information useful and informative. This is an excellent supplement that promotes health in many different ways. Use it effectively to treat some of the most unwanted physical conditions around today.

Thank You Page

I want to personally thank you for reading my book. I hope you found information in this book useful and I would be very grateful if you could leave your honest review about this book. I certainly want to thank you in advance for doing this.

www.ingramcontent.com/pod-product-compliance
Lightning Source LLC
Chambersburg PA
CBHW070342290526
45791CB00003B/1435